Summary

In 1993, President Clinton modified the military policy on providing abortions at military medical facilities. Under the change directed by the President, military medical facilities were allowed to perform abortions if paid for entirely with non-Department of Defense (DOD) funds (i.e., privately funded). Although arguably consistent with statutory language barring the use of Defense Department funds, the President's policy overturned a former interpretation of existing law barring the availability of these services. On December 1, 1995, H.R. 2126, the FY1996 DOD appropriations act, became law (P.L. 104-61). Included in this law was language barring the use of funds to administer any policy that permits the performance of abortions at any DOD facility except where the life of the mother would be endangered if the fetus were carried to term or where the pregnancy resulted from an act of rape or incest. Language was also included in the FY1996 DOD Authorization Act (P.L. 104-106, February 10, 1996) prohibiting the use of DOD facilities in the performance of abortions. These served to reverse the President's 1993 policy change. Recent attempts to change or modify these laws have failed.

Over the last three decades, the availability of abortion services at military medical facilities has been subjected to numerous changes and interpretations. Within the last 15 years, Congress has considered numerous amendments to effectuate such changes. Although Congress, in 1992, passed one such amendment to make abortions available at overseas installations, it was vetoed.

Abortions are generally not performed at military medical facilities in the continental United States. In addition, few have been performed at these facilities abroad for a number of reasons. First, the U.S. military follows the prevailing laws and rules of foreign countries regarding abortion. Second, the military has had a difficult time finding health care professionals in uniform willing to perform the procedure.

With the enactment of P.L. 104-61 and P.L. 104-106, these questions became moot, because now, neither DOD funds nor facilities may be used to administer any policy that provides for abortions at any DOD facility, except where the life of the mother may be endangered if the fetus were carried to term. Privately funded abortions at military facilities are permitted when the pregnancy was the result of an act of rape or incest.

In 2010, language was added to the Senate version of the FY2011 National Defense Authorization Act that would allow any DOD facilities to perform privately funded abortions. As noted, the military follows local laws and practices to the greatest extent possible. This potential change would not likely have much of an effect outside of the United States since nations that host large numbers of U.S. military personnel maintain legal restrictions on abortions. On September 21, 2010, and December 15, 2010, attempts were made to move this legislation to the Senate floor for a vote. However, due to disagreements over procedures, cloture votes were taken and failed. The House-passed version of this legislation does not contain language pertaining to abortion. The FY2011 National Defense Authorization Act became P.L. 111-383 without the Senate provision allowing military facilities to be used to perform abortions.

In 2011, attempts to expand coverage for cases of rape and incest and allow for privately funded abortion were blocked in the Senate.

Language in the Senate version of the National Defense Authorization Act for FY2013 would expand coverage of government-funded abortions for cases of rape and incest.

Contents

Tables

Appendixes

Contacts

Purpose

The purpose of this report is to describe and discuss the provisions for providing abortion services to military personnel, their dependents, and other military health care beneficiaries at military medical facilities. The report describes the history of these provisions, with particular emphasis on legislative actions. Finally, this report discusses a number of proposals to modify the law as well as other related legislative and administrative actions.

Issue

Language in the Senate version of the National Defense Authorization Act for FY2013 would expand coverage of government-funded abortions for cases of rape and incest.[1] Current law only allows for government-funded abortions in cases where the life of the mother would be at risk is the fetus was carried to term. Current law allows for privately funded abortion at military medical facilities where the life of the mother would be at risk is the fetus was carried to term or in cases where the pregnancy is the result of rape or incest.

Shortly after his inauguration on January 20, 1993, President Clinton issued a memorandum on abortions at military hospitals. This memorandum directed a change in policy so that abortions could be performed at military medical facilities provided that the procedure was "privately funded." This memo stated that:

> Section 1093 of title 10 of the United States Code prohibits the use of Department of Defense ("DOD") funds to perform abortions except where the life of a women would be endangered if the fetus were carried to term. By memorandum of December 21, 1987, and June 21, 1988, DOD has gone beyond what I am informed are the requirements of the statute and has banned all abortions at U.S. military facilities, even where the procedure is privately funded. The ban is unwarranted. Accordingly, I hereby direct that you reverse the ban immediately and permit abortion services to be provided, if paid for entirely with non-DOD funds and in accordance with other relevant DOD policies and procedures.[2]

The issue at hand was how the language in Title 10 of the United States Code and the President's memo were to be interpreted. As the President's memorandum made obvious, this language has been subject to varying interpretations that allowed or denied abortion services. Specifically, Section 1093 stated:

> Funds available to the Department of Defense may not be used to perform abortions except where the life of the mother would be endangered if the fetus were carried to term.[3]

---

[1] Cunningham, Paige Winfield, "Abortion Funding Fight Could Complicate Defense Spending Legislation," *The Washington Times*, May 30, 2012: 7.

[2] President William J. Clinton, Memorandum for the Secretary of Defense, Memorandum on Abortions in Military Hospitals, January 22, 1993; filed with the Office of the Federal Register, 11:50 a.m., January 27, 1993; cited in Public Papers of the Presidents of the United States, William J. Clinton, 1993, Washington, D.C., Government Printing Office, 1994: 11.

[3] 10 U.S.C. Sec. 1093, added P.L. 98-525, Sec. 1401(e)(5), October 19, 1984, 98 Stat. 2617. It should be noted that the Civilian Health and Medical Program of the Uniformed Services (CHAMPUS, now TRICARE), a medical program for military dependents, certain retirees and their dependents who are unable to receive care at a military medical facility, will provide coverage for abortions only when the mother's life is in danger. "The attending physician must certify in (continued...)

Although the President's interpretation of the language was arguably consistent with the letter of the law, critics contend that it countermanded the spirit of the statute and is overly broad. In other words, it is argued that the intent of this language was to prevent the DOD from providing abortion services. Proponents of the Clinton change argued that Congress allowed for exactly this type of interpretation. Proponents note that this interpretation was particularly important for eligible beneficiaries who are deployed overseas in areas where affordable and sanitary abortion services may not be available in the local economy.

Following the election of the 104th Congress, Democrats were replaced by Republicans as committee leaders. Representative Robert K. Dornan, the then-new Republican chairman of the Military Personnel and Compensation Subcommittee (the then-House National Security Committee), noted that one of his priorities "[was] barring abortions at overseas military hospitals, even if the patients pay for them."[4] On December 1, 1995, P.L. 104-61 was enacted. According to this law:

> Sec. 8119. None of the funds made available in this Act may be used to administer any policy that permits the performance of abortions at medical treatment or other facilities of the Department of Defense.
>
> Sec. 8119A. The provision of Section 8119 shall not apply where the life of the mother would be endangered if the fetus were carried to term, or the pregnancy is the result of an act of rape or incest.

On February 10, 1996, P.L. 104-106 was enacted. This law further limited that availability of abortion services:

> Sec. 738(b). RESTRICTION ON THE USE OF FACILITIES—No medical treatment facility or other facility of the Department of Defense may be used to perform an abortion except where the life of the mother would be endangered if the fetus were carried to term or in a case in which the pregnancy is the result of an act of rape or incest.[5]

Since then, efforts to modify the law pertaining to abortions have become a routine part of the legislative process. As noted above, language has been included in the Senate version of the FY2013 National Defense Authorization Act that would expand the availability of government-funded abortion to cases where the pregnancy was the result of rape and incest.

In conclusion, under current law, 10 U.S.C. Section 1093, Performance of Abortions: Restrictions

> (a) Restriction on Use of Funds.—Funds available to the Department of Defense may not be used to perform abortions except where the life of the mother would be endangered if the fetus were carried to term.

(...continued)

writing that the abortion was performed because a life-endangering condition existed, and must provide medical documentation to the CHAMPUS claims processor in order for CHAMPUS to share the cost of the procedure." See U.S. Department of Defense, OCHAMPUS, CHAMPUS Handbook, October 1994: 42.

[4] Maze, Rick, "Representative Dornan: 'Pay gap one of top concerns,'" *Army Times*, January 16, 1995: 3.

[5] U.S. Congress, Conference Committee, National Defense Authorization Act for Fiscal Year 1996, H.Rept. 104-450, S. 1124, 104th Cong., 2nd Sess., January 22, 1996: 206-207.

(b) Restriction on Use of Facilities.—No medical treatment facility or other facility of the Department of Defense may be used to perform an abortion except where the life of the mother would be endangered if the fetus were carried to term or in a case in which the pregnancy is the result of an act of rape or incest.

Background

There appears to be no evidence of a formal service policy on abortions prior to 1970. Sources familiar with the issue at that time note that the availability of abortion services at military medical facilities varied by service, location, physician, and "command milieu." Each of the services approached the issue differently. The Air Force tended to be somewhat more liberal, while the Army and the Navy tended to be somewhat more conservative. Each facility also tended to follow the laws and regulations of the state within which it was located. Individual physicians ultimately had a say regarding whether or not they personally would provide such services. Finally, the commanders of various medical facilities may have had some effect on how and under what circumstances abortion services may have been provided. Commanders often lead by example without explicitly stating their own opinions or policies, or giving direct orders. Subordinates are acutely aware of their commander's approach to issues and often will integrate this approach into their own practice. In other words, a policy may exist without one ever being officially stated. Although formal policy may not exist, physicians also follow professional guidelines, as they interpret them, by practicing "good medicine." Thus, the decision to provide an abortion may have been based on a host of medical indications particular to any given case. Generally, it appears that military physicians performed relatively few abortions at military medical facilities in this era.

In certain situations, such as in Vietnam (1961-1975), military medical facilities generally did not provide abortion services. Instead, medical evacuations to other countries that had available procedures (Japan, for example) provided access to abortion services.

In 1970, the office responsible for health affairs at DOD reportedly issued "orders that military hospitals perform abortions when it is medically necessary or when the mental health of the mother is threatened."[6] The rules, however, did not require military personnel to perform abortions. These rules were less restrictive than the abortion laws in a number of states. One year later, then-President Richard M. Nixon directed that military policy concerning abortions at military bases in the United States "be made to correspond with the laws of the States where the bases are located."[7] This correspondence of policy between the military and states (including foreign nations) came to be known as "the good neighbor policy."

---

[6] Wolffe, Jim, "Abortion ban may be lifted soon stateside," *Air Force Times*, April 12, 1993: 23.

[7] Statement about Policy on Abortions at Military Base Hospitals in the United States, April 3, 1971, Public Papers of the Presidents of the United States, Richard Nixon, 1971, Washington: GPO,1972) p. 500. Since CHAMPUS (the point of service contract health care for non-active duty beneficiaries—now known as TRICARE Standard) relied, then as now, on local health care providers, these individuals were already subject to State laws and regulations pertaining to abortion.

Following the 1973 Supreme Court case of *Roe v. Wade*,[8] the Department of Defense funded abortions for any women eligible for DOD health care, subject to certain limitations: first, two physicians were required to find that the abortion was "medically indicated" or required for "reasons of mental health"; second, the funding for these services could not be in conflict with the law of the state in which the abortion is carried out.[9] Since states had differing rules regarding abortion, it was possible for women to be treated differently depending on the location of the facility. Nevertheless, there remains anecdotal evidence of variations in accessibility similar to those that existed before *Roe v. Wade*.

In 1975, concerns were raised over inconsistencies between state statutes and the *Roe* decision. Military medical personnel were instructed to follow the constitutional guidance provided in *Roe* in certain instances, even though the state statutes had not been successfully challenged in court.[10]

From August 31, 1976, to August 31, 1977, approximately 26,000 abortions were performed in military hospitals or in the CHAMPUS program.[11]

In 1978, an amendment to the Department of Defense appropriations bill offered by Representative Robert Dornan prohibited the use of Defense Department funds for abortions with certain exceptions. This amendment, as enacted, stated that:

> None of the funds appropriated by this Act shall be used to perform abortions except where the life of the mother would be endangered if the fetus were carried to term; or except for such medical procedures necessary for the victims of rape or incest, when such rape or incest has been reported promptly to a law enforcement agency or public health service; or except in those instances where severe and long-lasting physical health damage to the mother would result if the pregnancy were carried to term when so determined by two physicians. Nor are payments prohibited for drugs or devices to prevent implantation of the fertilized ovum, or for medical procedures necessary for the termination of an ectopic pregnancy.[12]

In 1979, similar language was enacted in the FY1980 DOD appropriations act. The 1979 language did not contain any restrictions with regard to the "severe and long-lasting physical health damage to the mother that would result if the pregnancy were carried to term when so determined by two physicians." In other words, a determination that carrying the pregnancy to term would affect the physical health of a woman was not a basis for providing abortions under this language.[13]

This language did not prevent all abortions at military hospitals. Military hospitals overseas reportedly performed approximately 1,300 abortions in FY1979. These abortions were privately

---

[8] *Roe v. Wade*, 410 U.S. 113 (1973). The Court held that the Constitution protects a woman's decision whether or not to terminate pregnancy and that a State may not unduly burden the exercise of that fundamental right by regulations that prohibit or substantially limit access to the means of effectuating that decision.

[9] Ayres, B. Drummond, Jr., *New York Times*, August 10, 1978: 79 (microfilm).

[10] U.S. Department of Defense, Assistant Secretary of Defense (Health and Environment), James R. Cowen, Memorandum for the Assistant Secretaries of the Military Departments (M&RA), Abortion Policy, September 17, 1975.

[11] U.S. Department of Defense, Directorate for Defense Information, Press Division, 9 August, 1978.

[12] P.L. 95-457, §863, October 13, 1978, 92 Stat. 1254. In anticipation of this change, the Office of the Assistant Secretary of Defense (Public Affairs) published a News Release (September 29, 1978) functionally implementing this language effective September 30, 1978. This change also affected funding for CHAMPUS claims.

[13] P.L. 96-154, §762, December 21, 1979, 93 Stat. 1162.

paid for. Defense officials allowed these procedures under the rationale that at certain overseas (or isolated U.S.) stations, safe and reliable civilian facilities were not always available.[14]

In 1980, the language included in the FY1981 DOD appropriations act was again modified as follows:

> None of the funds appropriated by this Act shall be used to perform abortions except where the life of the mother would be endangered if the fetus were carried to term; or except for such medical procedures necessary for the victim of rape or incest, when such rape has within seventy-two hours been reported to a law enforcement agency or public health service; nor are payments prohibited for drugs or devices to prevent implantation of the fertilized ovum, or for medical procedures necessary for the termination of an ectopic pregnancy: *Provided, however,* That the several States are and shall remain free not to fund abortions to the extent that they in their sole discretion deem appropriate.[15]

Under this language, the reporting requirement for incest was removed. Also, victims of rape were required to report the incident within 72 hours.[16] In addition, language was added encouraging the states to exercise their authority with regard to funding abortions.

The language was shortened considerably in 1981. Many of the exceptions to the prohibition of funding were removed. This language stated that:

> None of the funds provided by this Act shall be used to perform abortions except where the life of the mother would be endangered if the fetus were carried to term.[17]

Identical language was included in the following two years' appropriations acts.[18] Finally, in 1984, Congress codified this language in Title 10, United States Code (see quoted text at the top of page 1).[19]

In 1988, DOD modified its rules to require a physician's statement for abortion claims made via CHAMPUS. This change was instituted to assure that all claims for abortions performed in the private sector and covered by CHAMPUS were for life-threatening situations. "CHAMPUS officials said life-threatening conditions include leukemia, breast cancer and other malignancies, kidney failure, congestive heart failure, severe heart disease, uncontrolled diabetes and several other conditions."[20]

On June 21, 1988, Dr. William Mayer, then-Assistant Secretary of Defense (Health Affairs), issued a memorandum barring abortions in military medical. Although Dr. Mayer recognized that

---

[14] Smith, Paul, "1300 FY79 O'seas Abortions Revealed," *Army Times*, December 8, 1980: 2.

[15] P.L. 96-527, §760, December 15, 1980, 94 Stat. 3091.

[16] Previous language required that such a report should be made "promptly." DOD interpreted this to mean within 48 hours. It was also expected that victims of incest would report the incident(s) to appropriate authorities, however, the lack of a time restriction meant that a report could be delayed indefinitely. (See "DOD Issues New Rules On Abortion," *Army Times*, March 9, 1981: 15.)

[17] P.L. 97-114, §757, December 29, 1981, 95 Stat. 1588.

[18] P.L. 97-377, §755, December 21, 1982, 96 Stat. 1860; P.L. 98-212, §751, December 8, 1983, 97 Stat. 1447.

[19] 10 U.S.C. 1093, P.L. 98-525, sec 1401(e)(5), October 19, 1984, 98 Stat. 2617. Note this change occurred via an authorization act and not as a part of the appropriations process (*Omnibus Defense Authorization Act, 1985*).

[20] Kimble, Vesta, "Doctor's Statement Needed for Abortion Claims," *Navy Times*, March 14, 1988: 24.

---

privately paid abortions did not violate the letter of the law, he issued the memorandum to avoid the appearance of "insensitivity to the spirit" of the law.[21]

In 1990, an attempt to overturn this restriction failed. An amendment (to the DOD authorization act) to allow abortions at military medical facilities overseas was withdrawn when the Senate fell two votes short of the number needed to invoke cloture (58-41).[22] The House of Representatives rejected a similar amendment.

On May 22, 1991, the House of Representatives reversed itself and passed (220-208) an amendment to the DOD authorization act that would have reinstated the pre-paid overseas policy. Proponents argued that the language would be merely a return to the policy as it existed prior to Dr. Mayer's memo of 1988. Opponents countered that, as drafted, the amendment offered by Representative AuCoin would go beyond the then-prevailing policy by allowing abortions for any reason and at any time during the pregnancy.[23] The measure was rejected once again when the Senate fell two votes short of the 60 votes needed to invoke cloture (58-40).[24]

The battle over this language intensified. Proponents stated that military women or dependents overseas were forced into dangerous or life-threatening situations in countries where safe, legal, or affordable abortions could not be provided. Opponents argued that no woman was denied military transportation to receive access to an abortion in another country.

Again in 1992, Representative AuCoin introduced language to overturn the restrictions on abortions at overseas military facilities. This amendment was passed (216-193).[25] On September 18, 1992, the Senate rejected (36-55) an effort to strike language overturning the restrictions on overseas abortions. Despite these votes, it was expected that President George H. W. Bush would veto any defense legislation reinstating the former policy. This expected veto was cited as the reason for the language being dropped by the conferees.[26] By unanimous consent, the Senate agreed to substitute the language pertaining to overseas abortions into S. 3144 after striking all after the enacting clause.[27] S. 3144 was simultaneously passed by unanimous consent. The House subsequently passed the measure (220-186) on October 3, 1992.[28]

---

[21] "Abortion Is Restricted At Military Hospitals," *New York Times*, July 19, 1988: A11. "The abortion issue in military hospitals has a symbolic and political importance that dwarfs the actual numbers of people involved. Military hospitals overseas performed only six abortions in the last year they were permitted [1987]." Willis, Grant, "Clinton Ends Ban on Military Abortions," *Air Force Times*, February 1, 1993: 4; and, U.S., Department of Defense, Assistant Secretary of Defense, William Mayer, M.D., Memorandum for Military Departments, DOD Policy Regarding Non-Funded Abortions in Outside the Continental United States Medical Treatment Facilities, June 21, 1988, "The policy is that the performance of pre-paid abortions in military treatment facilities is not authorized."

[22] Congressional Record, August 3, 1990: S11813-S11824.

[23] Congressional Record, May 22, 1991: H3394 et seq.

[24] Nelson, Soraya, "Overseas Abortion Amendment Fails," *Army Times* December 1991: 16.

[25] Congressional Record, June 4, 1992: H4150-H4156.

[26] Dewar, Helen, "Bush's Veto Power Stalled the Abortion-Rights Push in Congress," *Washington Post*, November 30, 1991: A6.

[27] Both House and Senate versions of the FY1993 Defense Authorization Act contained provisions that would "entitle military personnel and their dependents to reproductive health care services in a medical facility of the uniformed services outside the United States on a reimbursement basis.... The conferees agree to exclude this provision. The Senate has passed a bill (S. 3144) that contains this provision. The House intends to pass this bill and send it to the President as soon as possible." U.S. Congress, House Conference Committee, National Defense Authorization Act for Fiscal Year 1993, H.Rept. 102-966, H.R. 5006, 102d Cong., 2nd Sess., October 1, 1992: 716.

[28] See H.Res. 589, Congressional Record, October 2, 1992: H10803-H10804, and Congressional Record, October 3, (continued...)

Arguably, the Senate and House agreed to remove this language from the DOD authorization act in anticipation of a presidential veto. By removing the language and passing it as a free-standing bill, the authorization act was not jeopardized. Since this was not presented in the authorization act, it remains unknown whether President Bush would have exercised his veto authority over the entire bill. Nevertheless, President Bush did pocket-veto S. 3144 on October 31, 1992 (after the congressional adjournment). No attempt was made to override this veto.[29]

As a result of President Clinton's 1993 memorandum (see page 1), then-Secretary of Defense Les Aspin directed the secretaries of the military departments to reinstate the pre-1988 policy concerning the availability of abortions overseas. On May 9, 1994, the Assistant Secretary of Defense (Health Affairs), Dr. Stephen C. Joseph, released a memorandum[30] seeking to unify and make consistent DOD policy. This policy had five parts that (1) provided access to abortion services for service women and eligible dependents overseas, (2) required the valid consent of a parent or other designated person in the case of a minor who was "not mature enough and well enough informed to give valid consent," (3) relieved those medical practitioners directly involved from performing abortions if they objected, (4) respected host nation laws regarding abortion, and, (5) directed the Military Health Services System to provide other means of access if providing pre-paid abortion services at a facility was not feasible. Such alternate means could include supplementing staff with contract personnel, referrals, travel, etc. The cost of an abortion had been reported to be about $500.[31] (It should be noted that cost determination is not based on the actual cost of the service to the military but rather on estimates. As a result of the way DOD funds accounts, i.e., personnel, construction, operations and maintenance, etc., it is difficult to determine the valid cost of any one procedure. This has led some to question whether or not any federal funds are used in cases of "pre-paid" abortions.)

In practice, the policy instituted by President Clinton's 1993 action may not have had the effects the President had expected. Although abortion access had been liberalized in terms of overall policy, liberalization had not necessarily occurred in terms of actual access.

> In the six years preceding the 1988 ban, military hospitals overseas had performed an average of 30 abortions annually. Last spring, though, when the military medical officials surveyed 44 Army, Navy and Air Force obstetricians and gynecologists stationed in Europe, they found that all but one doctor adamantly refused to perform the procedure.
>
> That one holdout, too, quickly switched positions.... No military medical personnel willing to perform abortions have stepped forward in the Pentagon's sprawling Pacific theater of operations, either.[32]

A number of reasons have been advanced to explain this general unwillingness by health care personnel in uniform to perform these procedures. First, fewer medical schools require or provide training in these techniques than was the case in the years immediately following the *Roe v. Wade*

(...continued)

1992: H10966-H10975.

[29] Congressional Quarterly, December 19, 1992: 3926.

[30] U.S. Department of Defense, Assistant Secretary of Defense (Health Affairs), Memorandum, Implementation of Policy Regarding Pre-Paid Abortions in Military Treatment Facilities, May 9, 1994: 2p.

[31] Nelson, Soraya S., "Pentagon Pens Rules on Abortion," *Army Times*, May 23, 1994: 10.

[32] Morrison, David C., "An Order That Didn't Take," *National Journal*, April 16, 1994: 900.

decision.[33] Second, it is widely thought that the military in general, and military physicians in particular, tends to be more conservative on social issues than many population cohorts. Even if training were made available it is unlikely that many would volunteer. Third, the social order on military posts tends to be very close-knit and hierarchical. A subordinate may choose not to "ruffle the feathers" of a superior over such a contentious issue. Thus, the social norms established by superiors in the military environment are likely to translate into action or inaction by subordinates. This conventional wisdom gains credibility given the enormous amount of leverage superiors in the military have over the careers of subordinates. (Although this is true in the civilian context, it apparently exists to a lesser degree, especially in professional fields such as medicine in which civilians are generally unwilling to formally judge or second-guess professional colleagues.) Fourth, the medical team must consist of volunteers. Any member of a medical team needed to perform an abortion can essentially "veto" it. Fifth, since military physicians are paid a salary, and not on the basis of procedures performed, there is no economic incentive to provide abortions. Finally, rules exist requiring the services to respect the prevailing laws in each country. Thus, the restrictions of a particular country may limit the access to pre-paid abortions at military facilities (see **Appendix**).[34]

Given these factors and considerations, it was reported that 27 abortions were performed at military hospitals worldwide in 1993[35] and 10 in 1994. All of the 1994 abortions were reported to be "life of the mother" cases; that is, none were "pre-paid." According to data provided by the military services, the following table displays the number of therapeutic abortions by year by service:

Table 1. Therapeutic Abortions at Military Treatment Facilities

	1996	FY 97	FY 98	FY 99	FY 00	FY 01	FY 02	FY 03	FY 04	FY 05	FY 06	FY 07	FY 08	FY 09	TOTAL
Armya	4	3	1	1	0	4	4	3	3	4	1	2	3	1	34
Navyb									4	2	2	2	3	1	14
Air Forcec,d	1	1	0	1	0	1	0	0	0	0	1	0	0	0	5
TOTAL	5	4	1	2	0	5	4	3	7	6	4	4	6	2	53

Source: Department of Defense

Notes:

---

[33] According to the Alan Guttmacher Institute, from 1976 to 1991, the proportion of residency programs that did not offer abortion training rose from 7.5 to 31%. In 1976, 26% of the residency programs required abortion training. By 1991, only 12% required such training. The Accreditation Council for Graduate Medical Education has directed obstetrical residents should be taught how to perform abortions, unless they have a moral or religious objection. This change in policy was scheduled to become effective on January 1, 1996. Abortion mandated for OB training, *Washington Times*, February 15, 1995: A12. On March 19, 1996, the Senate passed the Coats amendment (no. 3513): "to amend the Public Health Service Act to prohibit governmental discrimination in the training and licensing of health professionals on the basis of the refusal to undergo or provide training in the performance of induced abortions," by a vote of 63 yeas and 37 nays. Congressional Record, March 19, 1996, S2262-S2266, S2268-S2276, S2280.

[34] "Most countries where American military personnel are stationed restrict or outlaw them [abortions] altogether." Nelson, Soraya S., "Limits Remain on Abortions at Overseas Hospitals," *Navy Times*, February 22, 1993: 11.

[35] Nelson, Soraya S., "Military Abortions Overseas: Still Rare," *Army Times*, September 5, 1994: 18.

a.   ICD-9 Code Ranges: 635-636. Data Source Standard Inpatient Data Record (SIDR). All cases have been reviewed and determined to be within compliance of Federal law.

b.   ICD-9 Code Ranges: 635-636. No encounters for 636. Data source is the Standard Inpatient Data Record (SIDR) in the MHS Mart (M2) database. Data in M2 is truncated at FY04 and historic data prior to FY04 is unavailable. MHS Coding Guide ines changed 1 July 2006; those cases identified before 2006 will be pulled and analyzed to insure that they were coded using the policies in place prior to the coding guide ine change.

c.   1996 is different because the only information available was one cover sheet/narrative summary/operation report on an Active Reserve member.

d.   Data from 1997 forward was retrieved from the Biometric Data Quality Assurance.

(Since 2010, DOD has not responded to CRS requests for data on abortions.)

Over these 15 years, DOD has performed an average of 3.79 therapeutic abortions per year.

Responding to the lack of medical personnel willing to perform abortions, the Army's 7th Medical Command (Europe) sought in 1993 to hire a civilian physician whose duties would include providing abortion services.[36] This move would have been consistent with the President's memo stating that "[i]n circumstances in which it is not feasible to provide pre-paid abortion services in a particular military facility, the [Military Health Services System] shall develop other means to assure access." Such an affirmative step would have provided access where none was available before. However, such a step could have been viewed as encouraging abortion and threatened to provoke protests both within the uniformed services and in the international community.[37] To date, reports of protests have not been found.

Another consideration along similar lines is to expand the use of foreign physicians, as suggested by the Defense Advisory Committee for Women in the Services (DACOWITS). This may be effective in certain situations, but not all, since DOD is still required, as a result of the "good neighbor policy," to observe local laws. Countries such as Spain, South Korea, and Panama outlaw or sharply restrict abortions.[38]

Following German unification, in 1993, a German court issued an injunction against a law that would have unified abortion policies in the east and west. The *Bundestag*, lower house of the German parliament, struggled to write new laws. During this void, the performance of abortions or restrictions on abortion services at military facilities in Germany, although not illegal, may have been inflammatory to certain German sensitivities.[39] On August 21, 1995, German President Roman Herzog signed into law a measure passed by the *Bundestag* (on June 29) and approved by the *Bundesrat*, upper house (on July 14). Under this law, abortions are illegal (except in cases of rape or "medical necessity"), but a woman who seeks an abortion during the first 12 weeks of

---

[36] Scholar, Steve, "Army Seeking Civilian Doctor Willing To Do abortions at Military Hospitals," *Stars and Stripes* (European), April 28, 1993: 1.

[37] "A Pentagon Decision To Send Doctors Overseas To Perform Abortions in Military Hospitals Could Spark Protest from Pro-Life Groups in Germany, Pro-Life GIs say," Pro-Life Protests, American Legion, July 1994: 10.

[38] "Women in the services," Fast Track, *Army Times*, July 4, 1994: 20.

[39] "Women's groups, opposition politicians from the west, and easterners across the political spectrum expressed outrage at the court's decision. Many observers felt the decision exposed the deep east-west social divide." CRS Issue Brief IB91018, *German-American Relations in the New Europe*, by Karen E. Donfried, January 27, 1994, p. 6 (out-of-print; available from the author at 7-8033).

pregnancy will not be subject to criminal prosecution provided she attends a compulsory counseling session reviewing her options.[40]

Contracting with foreign physicians poses its own problems. Countries that lack professional medical personnel trained to U.S. standards (the very reason argued for providing these services in the first place) are less likely to have physicians with a skill level that would be commendable for contracting.

In certain cases, contracting may be an option, but it raises other considerations. If the patient was to pay the cost of the abortion, does such a cost include a pro-rated amount based on contracting, training, travel, and other costs required to provide these services? Inclusion of these in such a cost calculation could well make the price of these services prohibitive. Conversely, using Defense Department funds to make available "pre-paid" abortions (i.e., through contracting, travel, etc.) could be viewed as in conflict with 10 U.S.C. 1093.

According to a DOD Information Paper, in August 1994, "a policy on hiring non-military physicians to perform abortions was issued with specific reference to treatment facilities in Germany. DOD respects host nation laws regarding abortion."[41]

Furthermore, it was unlikely that abortion services would become more available if the military reduced the number of physicians as part of downsizing of the force structure. One drawdown proposal suggests that DOD could reduce the number of physicians in uniform by as much as 50%.[42] Under the Administration's long-term defense spending plans, 5,600 civilian medical personnel will be cut from the Army over the next six years. The Navy and Air Force, together, are expected to be reduced by less than 2,000. These reductions "amount to the equivalent of shutting three of the Army's eight medical centers, experts say."[43] The reduction of civilian professionals in the U.S. military may require DOD to rotate uniformed physicians back to the United States from overseas, further reducing the number of physicians overseas. Such a reduction would likely serve to reduce the availability of abortion services overseas.

On May 29, 2002, a federal judge ruled that the military must pay for a 1994 abortion of an anencephalic fetus.[44] Later, in August 2002, a second federal court ruled likewise in a separate case involving another anencephalic fetus.[45] Both cases were reversed on appeal.[46]

---

[40] *The Week in Germany*, January 30, 1998.

[41] Memorandum for Assistant Secretary of Defense (Health Affairs), Information Paper on abortion policy for Dr. Hambre's confirmation hearing, July 1997.

[42] "In June [1994], a Pentagon study found that only about half of the current number of military doctors are needed for any foreseeable military operation." Jowers, Karen, "50% Cut Is Planned in Military Doctors," *Air Force Times*, January 23, 1995: 28.

[43] Nelson, Soraya S., "Medicare Users May Lose Hospital Access," *Navy Times*, September 5, 1994: 26.

[44] *Britell v. United States*, 204 F.Supp.2d 182, May 29, 2002.

[45] Ostrom, Carol M., "Judge: Navy Must Cover Women's Abortion," *Seattle Times*, August 13, 2002. The 9th Circuit Court of Appeals, without comment, denied a last minute appeal in this case. "Court Rejects Effort to Stop Navy Funding of Abortion," *Baltimore Sun*, August 18, 2002.

[46] *Britell v. United States*, 372 F.3d 1370, June 24, 2004, and *Doe v. USA*, et al., civil docket for case #: 2:02-cv-01657-TSZ, August 18, 2005.

"Plan B" and RU-486

In February 2002, the DOD Pharmacy and Therapeutics (P&T) Executive Council recommended adding levonorgestrel, aka "Plan B," to the Basic Core Formulary,[47] subject to further review. Plan B is described as an emergency contraceptive used to prevent pregnancy following a known or suspected contraceptive failure (e.g., broken condom) or when a pregnancy may result because no contraception was used (e.g., rape). It is noted that it will not terminate an "established pregnancy." In other words, it is not RU-486, a known abortifacient, which chemically induces an abortion. RU-486 is subject to restrictions under 10 U.S.C. Section 1093.[48]

According to a DOD Information Paper, Plan B could possibly "prevent a pregnancy by interfering with ovulation, sperm transport through cervical mucus and fallopian tubes, release of pituitary gonadotropins, corpus luteum functions, fertilization, *embryo transport and implantation.*"[49] [emphasis added] The possibility of preventing a fertilized egg from implanting leads to the argument, for those who maintain that life begins at conception, that Plan B represents a potential form of abortion in certain cases. In May 2002, the P&T Executive Council Meeting released the following:

> At the February 2002 DOD Pharmacy & Therapeutics (P&T) Executive Council meeting, the Council recommended the addition of levonorgestrel 0.75 mg (Plan B) to the Basic Core Formulary (BCF), subject to the review of the Director, TRICARE Management Activity (TMA) and/or the Assistance Secretary of Defense for Health Affairs (ASD(HA)). On 28 March 2002, the Executive Director of TMA signed an Action Memo approving the recommendation. On April 3, 2002 the co-chair of the DOD P&T Committee informed the Council members and pharmacy consultants of the decision, and re-informed the Council on 7 May 2002. On 8 May 2002 the Executive Council was reconvened briefly to announce that the Council co-chairs had been informed that the ASD(HA) also wanted to review the Council's recommendation and that the Executive Director of TMA had rescinded his earlier approval. Therefore, Plan B has NOT been approved for addition to the BCF at this time, and the ASD(HA) is reviewing the Council's recommendation. [Military Treatment Facilities] MTFs are required to include all BCF drugs on their local formularies. As a result of Plan B's removal from the BCF, each MTF's P&T committee must now re-evaluate whether this product is within the scope of practice at the MTF and whether the MTF wants to continue to have Plan B on its formulary.[50]

In May 2005, a proposed amendment to make Plan B available on all military bases died in the House Rules Committee (as part of its consideration of the FY2005 National Defense Authorization Act).[51] This is not to say that Plan B was not available at certain military bases or to military health care beneficiaries. On September 7, 2005, it was reported that certain military

---

[47] The Basic Core Formulary or BCF refers to those pharmaceuticals that DOD makes available at DOD pharmacies.

[48] Legislation was offered in the 109th Congress (S. 511, Senator DeMint, March 3, 2005 and H.R. 1079, Rep. Bartlett) "To provide that the approved application under the Federal Food, Drug, and Cosmetic Act for the drug commonly known as RU-486 is deemed to have been withdrawn, to provide for the review by the Comptroller General of the United States of the process by which the Food and Drug Administration approved such drug, and for other purposes." Both bills were referred to Committees and have received no further action.

[49] Col. Daniel Remund, Co-chair, DOD Pharmacy & Therapeutics Committee, Information Paper, April 11, 2002.

[50] Department of Defense, Pharmaeconomic Center, Minutes of the DOD Pharmacy & Therapeutics Executive Council Meeting, May 7, 2002, pp. 2-3.

[51] The proposal was similar to language contained in H.R. 2635, Rep. Michael H. Michaud, May 25, 2005.

---

bases do have Plan B on hand and have offered it, usually in cases of sexual assault, but also in cases where other contraceptives failed or unprotected sex was involved. Further, military physicians may prescribe the medication allowing the beneficiary to have the prescription filled at civilian pharmacies.[52]

Although tangentially relevant to DOD policy, Plan B was the subject of controversy within the Food and Drug Administration (FDA):

> FDA Commissioner Lester Crawford on August 26 [2005] said the agency is indefinitely deferring Barr Laboratories' application for nonprescription sales of its emergency contraceptive Plan B and opening a 60-day public comment period on the application sparking charges that the decision was motivated by politics rather than science, ... FDA in May 2004 issued a "not approvable" letter in response to Barr's original application to allow Plan B – which can prevent pregnancy if taken within 72 hours of sexual intercourse – to be sold without a doctor's prescription and in January delayed a ruling on Barr's revised application, which would allow EC to be sold without a doctor's prescription only to women ages 17 and older. During a confirmation hearing in March, Crawford told the Senate committee that FDA would approve the application "within weeks."[53]

On August 24, 2006, the FDA approved over-the-counter sales of Plan B to women 18 years old and older.[54] Nearly three months later, Plan B began appearing in drug stores.[55]

Although this latter controversy was not directly related to the Department of Defense, it appears that the decision made by the FDA was taken into consideration by DOD officials with regard to emergency contraceptives.

In 2007, according to the DOD Pharmacoeconomic Center, Plan B was not on the Basic Core Formulary, but Military Treatment Facilities may have had it on hand as part of their formulary.[56]

In June 2009, Plan B was voluntarily discontinued by the manufacturer and replaced by a product under the name "Next Choice."

In November 2009, P&T Committee recommended placing Next Choice on the BCF. On February 3, 2010, this recommendation was approved by TMA and Next Choice was placed on the list of drugs all military facilities stock.[57]

---

[52] Montgomery, Nancy, Army Hospitals in Europe Offering 'Morning-After' Pill, *Stars and Stripes* (European edition), June 8, 2005.

[53] "FDA: Indefinitely Defers Decision on Emergency Contraceptive; Plan B," *National Journal Group, Inc.*, September 6, 2005

[54] Harris, Gardiner, F.D.A. Approves Broader Access t Next-Day Pill, *New York Times*, August 25, 2006: 1.

[55] Payne, January W., "For Plan B, A Broader Reach," *Washington Post*, November 21, 2006: F1.

[56] DOD, MTF Formulary Management For Contraceptives (Updated 26 Jan 07).

[57] Stein, Rob, "Pentagon to stock health facilities with morning-after pill," *The Washington Post*, February 5, 2010.

"Parental Notification"

"Parental notification" is concerned with those instances in which an abortion is sought at a military facility by or on behalf of a military dependent who is a minor and/or incapable of making such a decision.

According to DOD:

> Assuming that an abortion is authorized [under statute], consent must be obtained before any surgical procedure is performed. The requirement to obtain consent is required in military treatment facilities (MTFs), because the standard of care for medical practice in MTFs within the United States is governed by the Federal Tort Claims Act (FTCA). The standard of care for obtaining consent under FTCA is that the provider will follow state law governing the circumstances under which a minor may consent for medical treatment. In overseas facilities, consent by minors for abortions is governed by [DOD] Health Affairs Policy dated May 9, 1994, as amended by [DOD] Health Affairs Policy 96-030, dated February 13, 1996. Those policies state that the host nation laws or legal requirements will apply. In the absence of such host nation laws or legal requirements, valid consent for minors may be obtained in either of two methods. First, the consent of at least one parent or guardian is provided. Second, the commanding officer of the medical treatment facility (or if the commanding officer is not a physician, a senior physician designated by the commanding officer) makes a judgment, upon the recommendation of the attending physician, that the minor is mature enough and well enough informed to give valid consent, or, if she is not sufficiently mature and informed, that the desired abortion would be in her best interest.[58]

Legislative Action Since 1995

The House version of the FY1996 Defense Authorization Act contained a section that would terminate the policy of allowing the performance of abortions on a pre-paid basis, at military facilities. Under this language:

> This section would amend Section 1093 of Title 10, United States Code, to include restricting the Department of Defense from using medical treatment facilities or other DOD facilities, as well as DOD funds, to perform abortions unless necessary to save the life of the mother.[59]

The Senate report contained no similar provisions.

As a result of numerous political differences between the House and the Senate language, as well as Administration opposition on a number of issues raising the specter of a veto, the authorization act stalled in conference. Legislators sought to have language included in the FY1996 DOD appropriations act that would prohibit abortions at overseas military facilities. The Appropriations Conference Committee originally included the following language:

---

[58] Letter from Speight, Cynthia, CIV, OASD(HA)TMA to Richard Best, CRS, May 28, 2003.

[59] U.S. Congress, House Committee on National Security, *National Defense Authorization Act for Fiscal Year 1996*, H.Rept. 104-131, H.R. 1530, 104th Cong., 1st Sess., June 1, 1995: 237.

> Sec. 8119. None of the funds made available in this Act may be used to administer any policy that permits the performance of abortions at medical treatment or other facilities of the Department of Defense, except when it is made known to the federal official having authority to obligate or expend such funds that the life of the mother would be endangered if the fetus were carried to term: Provided, That the provisions of this section shall enter into force if specifically authorized in the National Defense Authorization Act for Fiscal Year 1996.

Thus, the nature of this language only allowed it to take effect, when and if the authorization language was enacted into law. As noted, at the time, the authorization bill was stalled in conference and faced a possible veto. The failure of the authorization bill to be passed would negate any language concerning abortions in the appropriations bill.

On September 29, 1995, pro-life legislators in the House and a large number of Democrats (opposed to the bill on policy and other spending considerations) joined ranks and rejected the conference version of the FY1996 DOD appropriations act (151-267), thereby returning the bill to the House-Senate conference.[60] On November 16, 1995, the conferees agreed to a compromise that included the following language:

> Sec. 8119. None of the funds made available in this Act may be used to administer any policy that permits the performance of abortions at medical treatment or other facilities of the Department of Defense.

> Sec. 8119A. The provision of Section 8119 shall not apply where the life of the mother would be endangered if the fetus were carried to term, or the pregnancy is the result of an act of rape or incest.

On December 1, 1995, the appropriations act, with the above two sections, became law.[61]

On December 15, 1995, the House passed the FY1996 Authorization Act (containing the language cited on page 13). The bill was approved by the Senate on December 19, 1995. On December 28, 1995, the President vetoed the authorization act, and in a letter to Congress, he stated:

> H.R. 1530 [FY1996 Defense Authorization Act] also contains ... provisions that would unfairly affect certain service members.... I remain very concerned about provisions that would restrict service women and female dependents of military personnel from obtaining privately funded abortions in military facilities overseas, except in the cases of rape, incest, or danger to the life of the mother. In many countries, these U.S. facilities provide the only accessible, safe source for these medical services. Accordingly, I urge Congress to repeal a similar provision that became law in the "Department of Defense appropriations act, 1996.[62]

On January 3, 1996, the House of Representatives failed to override the veto with a vote of 240-156. Two days later, the House amended S. 1124 by striking "all after the enacting clause of S. 1124 and insert[ing] in lieu thereof the text of H.R. 1530 [the vetoed language] as reported by the

---

[60] Maze, Rick, and William Matthew, "Defense Spending Bill Slapped Back by Unlikely Union in Congress," *Army Times*, October 9, 1995: 25.

[61] P.L. 104-61, 109 Stat. 636, December 1, 1995.

[62] Veto message from the President of the United States (H. Doc. No. 104-155), cited in the Congressional Record, January 3, 1996: H12.

committee of conference on December 13, 1995, contained in [H. Rept. 104-406]."[63] Under unanimous consent, the language was taken from the Speaker's table, as amended, and sent to conference. On January 22, conference report H.Rept. 104-450 was filed. On January 24, 1996, the House agreed to the conference report (287-129). Two day later, the Senate agreed to the conference report (56-34). Provisions barring the use of DOD facilities to perform abortions, except in cases of rape, incest or where the life of the mother would be endangered if the fetus were carried to term or in a case in which the pregnancy, were included in this language (see quoted text on page 2). On February 10, 1996, President Clinton signed the FY1996 Defense Authorization Act into law.[64]

Although the prohibition against using funding in the appropriations act would have lapsed at the end of the fiscal year, the change made via the authorization act modifies Title 10 United States Code. As such, this change will not lapse at the end of the fiscal year. Thus, this language will stay in effect unless and until Congress (with the President's signature) specifically acts to amend, modify, strengthen or repeal these provisions.

On May 14, 1996, an amendment was offered to the House version of the FY1997 National Defense Authorization Act to overturn the prohibition on military facilities performing abortions and allow such abortions to be performed at these medical facilities so long as federal funds are not used (i.e., patient-paid abortions). The amendment was defeat by a vote of 192 ayes and 225 noes.[65] Slightly more than one month later, the Senate passed an identical amendment to its version of the FY1997 National Defense Authorization Act by a voice vote.[66] Ultimately, the Senate conferees receded and the Senate amendment was dropped.

Efforts to amend these provisions have continued. On June 19, 1997, Representative Jane Harman offered an amendment to the FY1998 DOD Authorization Act that would purportedly

> [restore the] policy affording access to certain health care procedures for female members of the armed forces and dependents at Department of Defense facilities.

The amendment was rejected (196-224).[67]

In 1998, the House National Security Committee rejected another attempt to allow for privately funded abortions at these facilities.[68] On June 25, 1998, the Senate rejected a similar provision (44-49).[69]

During consideration of the FY2000 National Defense Authorization Act, the House Personnel Subcommittee accepted an amendment by Representative Loretta Sanchez to reverse the restrictions on privately funded abortions being performed at overseas military medical facilities. Another amendment, by Representative Kuykendall, would have allowed Defense Department funding of abortions in cases of rape or incest. Upon consideration by the House Armed Services

---

[63] Congressional Record, January 5, 1996: H302.

[64] P.L. 104-106, 110 Stat. 186, February 10, 1996.

[65] Congressional Record, May 14,1996, H5013-H5022.

[66] Congressional Record, June 19, 1996, S6460-S6469.

[67] Congressional Record, June 19, 1997, H4056-H4069.

[68] CQ Weekly, Other Policy Issues, May 9, 1998: 1240.

[69] Congressional Record, June 25, 1998, S7060-S7076.

Committee, the Sanchez amendment was dropped and the Kuykendall amendment was further amended by Representative Buyer. As amended, the Kuykendall amendment would allow Defense Department funding of abortions in cases of *forcible* rape or incest *provided that the rape or incest had been reported to a law enforcement agency.* [Italics represent the Buyer changes.] Later efforts to reinstate the Sanchez language allowing for abortions at overseas military facilities when personal funds are used were rejected by both the House and the Senate. Ultimately, the Kuykendall amendment, as amended, was also deleted during conference consideration of the FY2000 National Defense Authorization Act, thereby leaving the law unchanged.[70]

Although not specifically related to the above discussion of the military abortion issue, other language has been proposed that would have had an effect on the consideration of the abortion issue. H.R. 2436[71] included, in part, language modifying Title 10, United States Code. According to this language, any conduct violating certain provisions of the Uniform Code of Military Justice, by a person subject to the Uniform Code of Military Justice, that causes death or bodily injury to a fetus who is in utero at the time the conduct takes place, would be guilty of a criminal offense. For example, if during an assault on a pregnant women, the fetus were injured, such an injury would constitute a separate offense. Exceptions were included in cases of abortions, medical treatment of the woman, or conduct of the woman with regard to her fetus. On September 30, 1999, the House passed this language (254-172). The next day, it was received and read in the Senate. On February 23, 2000, the Senate Committee on Judiciary held hearings on a Senate companion bill, S. 1673. No further action was then taken by the Senate, and the legislation failed to become law. (Similar language was considered in 2004; see "Unborn Victims of Violence Act 2004," below.)

Proponents note that such language would recognize the victimization of the child while in utero and afford appropriate criminal sanctions to perpetrators of violent acts. Critics view the inclusion of such language as a means of defining a fetus as a victim and thereby acknowledging or creating a separate human existence. These critics are concerned that such language would arguably recognize the fetus as separate person in the eyes of the law thereby complicating the abortion debate.[72]

In consideration of the FY2001 National Defense Authorization Act (H.R. 4205), the House Armed Services Committee "voted to retain its ban on abortions at military hospitals unless the mother's life is at risk. The 31-20 vote came May 10, 2000, on an amendment that would have allowed abortions at overseas hospitals if patients rather than the government paid for them. The 29-26 vote came on a failed try to allow military hospitals to perform abortions in cases of rape or incest."[73] Eight days later, a floor amendment was offered that would strike subsections a and b of 10 U.S.C. Section 1093, effectively removing any restriction to providing abortions under this title. The amendment was defeated (221-195).[74]

---

[70] Maze, Rick, "Abortion Provision Dropped from Defense Bill," *Times*, August 16, 1999: 11.

[71] H.R. 2436, Representative Linsey Graham, July 1, 1999.

[72] For additional information on the legal aspects of the abortion issue, see CRS Report RL33467, *Abortion Judicial History and Legislative Response*, by Jon O. Shimabukuro.

[73] FastTrack, *Times*, May 29, 2000: 6.

[74] Congressional Record, May 18, 2000: H3347-H3350, H3371.

On June 20, 2000, the Senate tabled (50-49) an amendment to the FY2001 National Defense Authorization Act, S. 2549, that would strike Section b of 10 U.S.C. Section 1093. The amendment would have lifted the ban on the use of military facilities in performing abortions. Although proponents noted that the amendment "would lift restrictions on privately funded abortions at military facilities overseas," as written, the amendment would affect such facilities in the United States as well.[75]

On September 25, 2001, Representative Loretta Sanchez offered an amendment to the National Defense Authorization Act for FY2002. This amendment would have limited the restriction on the use of DOD facilities for performing abortions at those facilities "in the United States." In other words, this language would remove the restriction of providing privately funded abortion services at DOD facilities overseas. The amendment was rejected (199-217).[76]

During debate on the Bob Stump FY2003 National Defense Authorization Act, the Senate (52-40) passed an amendment that would remove the restriction on the use of military facilities.[77] The House had earlier rejected a similar measure (215-202).[78] In a letter to Senator Carl Levin, then-Chairman of the Armed Services Committee, Secretary of Defense Donald H. Rumsfeld wrote:

> The Senate bill removes the current statutory prohibition on access to abortion services at Department of Defense (DOD) medical facilities. The President's senior advisors would recommend that the President veto the bill if it changes current law.[79]

The Senate amendment was dropped by the conference committee.[80]

On April 1, 2004, President Bush signed H.R. 1997, "Unborn Victims of Violence Act of 2004 (Laci and Conner's Law)" into law.[81] Although intended to protect fetuses, this legislation contains a provision that would not permit the prosecution "of any person for conduct relating to an abortion" in which consent was legally obtained or implied.

Amendments to the FY2004 National Defense Authorization Act to modify the law were also offered. In the House, an amendment that would have limited the restriction on DOD facilities to the United States was rejected (201-227).[82]

Likewise the Senate rejected (48-51) an amendment that would have repealed the restriction on using DOD facilities, in general.[83]

However, the Senate agreed, subject to certain limitations, to consider legislation, S. 1104,[84] "to provide for parental involvement in abortions of dependent children of the Armed Forces." The legislation was placed on the Legislative Calendar[85] but failed to be called to the floor.

---

[75] Congressional Record, June 20, 2000: S5406-S5421, S5425.

[76] Congressional Record, September 25, 2001: H6022-25, H6032-33.

[77] Congressional Record, June 21, 2002: S5882.

[78] Congressional Record, May 9, 2002: H2380.

[79] Letter from Secretary of Defense Donald H. Rumsfeld to the Honorable Carl Levin, September 24, 2002.

[80] Congressional Record, November 12, 2002: H8462.

[81] P.L. 108-212; 1185 Stat. 568; April 1, 2004.

[82] Congressional Record, May 22, 2003: H4571.

[83] Congressional Record, May 22, 2003: S6911.

Consideration of the Ronald W. Reagan FY2005 National Defense Authorization Act included a number of amendments regarding abortion services. In the House of Representatives, Representative Susan A. Davis introduced an amendment that would allow military personnel and their dependents to use their own funds to obtain abortion services at overseas military hospitals. This amendment was defeated (202-221).[86]

In the Senate, an amendment offered by Senator Barbara Boxer, would allow DOD funding of abortions in cases of rape or incest. This amendment, along with 25 other amendments, was passed *en bloc* by unanimous consent.[87] On October 8, 2004, the conference report for this legislation noted that the "Boxer amendment" had been dropped.[88]

Two other Senate amendments to the Ronald W. Reagan FY2005 National Defense Authorization Act (H.R. 4200) were submitted. The first, S.Amdt. 3406 (Senators Frist and Brownback), would "provide for parental involvement in the performance of abortions for dependent children of members of the Armed Forces." The second, S.Amdt. 3407 (Senators Frist and Brownback), would require the notification of authorities regarding the identity of perpetrators, where possible, in cases of rape or incest when abortions are sought at military facilities. Neither S.Amdt. 3406 nor S.Amdt. 3407 was called up.

On May 25, 2005, the House of Representatives considered an amendment (offered by Representative Susan Davis) to the National Defense Authorization Act for Fiscal Year 2006 (H.R. 1815). The amendment would allow overseas military facilities to provide privately funded abortions for women who are in the miliary or are military dependents. This amendment was rejected (194-233).[89]

On July 25, 2005, Senator Lautenberg filed an amendment in the Senate that would "restore the previous policy regarding restrictions on the use of medical treatment facilities or other Department of Defense facilities." This amendment would strike Section 1093(b) of title 10 U.S.C. (and remove the title language "Restriction on Use of Funds.–" from Section 1093(a)). No further action has been taken on this amendment.[90]

On May 10, 2006, the House of Representatives considered an amendment (offered by Representative Robert E. Andrews) to the John Warner FY2007 National Defense Authorization Act that would allow overseas military facilities to provide privately funded abortions for women who are in the military or are military dependents. This amendment was rejected (191-237).

(...continued)

[84] Senator Brownback, May 22, 2003.

[85] Congressional Record, May 22, 2003: D576. See also, "Congress Votes to Keep the Abortion Ban on Bases," *Washington Post*, May 23, 2003: A7.

[86] Congressional Record, May 19, 2004: H3358.

[87] Congressional Record, June 22, 2004: S7152.

[88] Congressional Record, October 8, 2004: H9549.

[89] Congressional Record, May 25, 2005: H4009-H4013, H4017.

[90] Congressional Record, July 25, 2005, S8845.

Recent Legislative Action

Language included in the Senate version of the National Defense Authorization Act for Fiscal Year 2011[91] would, if enacted, repeal the prohibition on using any military facilities to perform abortion, with certain exceptions. This action would allow the Department of Defense to return to the Clinton administration policy of allowing military facilities to provide abortions using private funds. Similar language was not included in the House version. On September 21, 2010, and December 15, 2010, attempts were made to move this legislation to the floor for a vote. However, due to disagreements over procedures, cloture votes were taken and failed. Ultimately, the FY2011 National Defense Authorization Act became P.L. 111-383 without the Senate provision allowing military facilities to be used to perform abortions.

Amendments to the National Defense Authorization Act for FY 2012, offered by Sen. Jeanne Shaheen, were not include in the final passed version. S.Amdt. 1120 would have expanded government-funded abortion at military medical facilities to include pregnancies resulting from rape or incest. S.Amdt. 1121 would have removed subsection 10 U.S.C. 1093(b) thereby allowing for a return to the Clinton policy of allowing privately funded abortions.[92]

As noted on page 1, it was reported that language had been included in the National Defense Authorization Act for FY 2013 that would allow for government-funded abortions in cases where the pregnancies resulted from rape or incest.

---

[91] U.S. Congress, Senate, Armed Services Committee, National Defense Authorization Act for Fiscal Year 2011, S.Rept. 111-201, S. 3454, 111th Cong., 2nd Sess., June 4, 2010: 149.

[92] P.L. 112-81, SA 1120 was determined to be nongermane and SA 1121 was submitted on Nov. 17, 2011, with no further action listed in LIS.

Appendix. Availability of Abortion Services at Military Facilities Overseas

According to Department of Defense and individual command officials (as reported to the *Army Times*, September 5, 1994: 18; source: Defense Department and individual command officials), the availability of abortion services (prior to the restrictions enacted on December 1, 1995) at military facilities overseas could vary depending on location.

GERMANY

- **National policy:** See discussion on page 9 above.

- **Local U.S. military policy:** Under German law, abortions are illegal except in cases of rape or medical necessity. Abortions carried out during the first twelve weeks of pregnancy are not considered a prosecutable offense provided the woman has certification attesting to receiving state approved counseling to review her options. The military does not allow abortions at its facilities.

- **Since the U.S. ban was lifted:** Estimates of how many American service women or family members received abortions from German providers in 1993 are as high as 1,500, although German officials say there is no way to confirm this number.

ITALY

- **National policy:** Abortions are permitted. They must be performed by a licensed gynecologist.

- **Local U.S. military policy:** Abortion services comparable to those in the United States are available from Italian providers in the Naples and Sigonella areas. Service women and family members who desire abortions are referred to pre-identified licensed local providers. Abortions are not performed at military hospitals.

- **Since the U.S. ban was lifted:** One elective abortion was reportedly provided in Sigonella at an Italian facility.

JAPAN

- **National policy:** Abortion is legal and fairly unrestricted, but more expensive than in the United States.

- **Local U.S. military policy:** Given that abortions are readily available in the Japanese community, women seeking abortion from Navy hospitals here are referred to family-service counselors for referrals to Japanese doctors.

- **Since the U.S. ban was lifted:** Few, if any, abortions were performed at military hospitals, Navy officials said. The number of abortions by civilian doctors is unknown.

KOREA

- **National policy:** Abortion is illegal except to save the life of the mother. However, it has been noted that Korean women have not been denied access to medically provided abortion services despite this law.

- **Local U.S. military policy:** The U.S. military's rules for Korea could not be learned from military officials, but because of the local law, abortions would not be available at U.S. hospitals. However, since Korean women have access to such services, it is reasonable to infer that such services could also be available to U.S. service women off-base.

- **Since the U.S. ban was lifted:** Service members or family members continue to have to travel outside of Korea to obtain an abortion.

For a country-by-country listing of abortion laws and policies go to the following website: http://www.un.org/esa/population/publications/abortion/profiles.htm.

Problematic Comparisons to Foreign Military Policies

Abortion policies of foreign militaries vary. These variations depend on the country's general policy regarding abortion. For instance, abortion policies are affected by religion (Vatican, Israel, and Islamic nations, for example), population control policies (China) and other cultural factors (nationalized health care policies, such as are found in Great Britain), and issues pertaining to the structure of the military—the presence of women in uniform (many Islamic countries do not have women in uniform, making the issue moot). Some countries do not have a military (Costa Rica for instance does not have a military per se but rather a paramilitary style security force). In addition, internal legal restrictions or rulings, such as court rulings on abortion (see Germany), affect the country's policy. Finally, very few countries maintain a level of overseas deployments that make direct comparisons relevant. For these reasons, comparisons to foreign nations in terms of their abortion policy in general, and their policy regarding military abortions at overseas military medical facilities, in particular, are difficult to justify and of questionable utility.

Author Contact Information

David F. Burrelli
Specialist in Military Manpower Policy
dburrelli@crs.loc.gov, 7-8033

www.ingramcontent.com/pod-product-compliance
Lightning Source LLC
Chambersburg PA
CBHW081421170526
45166CB00010B/3424